ALDARA IMIQUIMOD USAGE GUIDE

What You Need to Know About Using Aldara Safely and Effectively for Skin Disorders

Dr. Garay Yusuf

Contents

CHAPTER ONE
The Quiet Giant of Topical Treatments

In the late 1980s, pharmaceutical researchers were looking for a way to help the body's immune system tackle certain skin conditions. That's when they came upon the small molecule that was to work wonders: Imiquimod. Unlike other creams, this one wasn't fighting the condition. It wasn't just killing bacteria or curing a virus outright; it was giving your body's natural defense system a boost to take over the fight.

Aldara, as it would later be marketed, wasn't a typical topical treatment. In its method of action, it aimed at kick-starting the body's immune cells by telling them, "You need to wake up and start attacking those cells that cause you trouble." That's the power of Imiquimod.

An Immune Boost – How Aldara Gets to Work

When you apply Aldara to the skin, it goes deep beneath the surface, triggering immune cells to start their work. More specifically, Imiquimod interacts with a protein called TLR7 on immune cells, or Toll-like receptor 7. It stimulates this receptor to kick-start an immune response, involving your body's own T-cells to recognize and destroy infected or abnormal cells.

Think of it this way: the cream isn't doing the work for you;

instead, it's sending up a flare to help get your immune system on the scene to start doing what needs to be done. For that reason, it is also known as an immune response modifier.

Genital Warts – A Tricky Condition Gets a Game-Changer

By the time Aldara hit the markets, one of the most famous uses was its treatment for genital warts, which were caused by the human papillomavirus known as

HPV. Genital warts are also notorious for being resistant to many over-the-counter and prescription means, many of which target the wart directly or use damage to the surrounding tissue to eradicate the infection. In contrast, Aldara wasn't like other treatments at all: it didn't harm healthy tissue. Instead, it amped up the body's immune response to recognize the wart as an invader.

The point is, consider the experience from the patient's perspective. Consider this woman fighting these warts for months or even years, trying everything from cryotherapy to laser treatments, with no success, until she's using Aldara's cream, which is not really taking care of the wart-it initiates a response; over these weeks of treatment, the immune system of this person starts to destroy the growth.

A Skin Cancer Alley – Helping Fight Superficial Basal Cell Carcinoma

But it wasn't just for warts. One of the most remarkable uses of Aldara is its role in treating superficial basal cell carcinoma (BCC), a form of skin cancer. Unlike its more aggressive cousin, squamous cell carcinoma, BCC tends to stay confined to the outer layers of the skin, making it treatable with topical interventions.

But for those who do not want to go under the knife, or whose cancer has infiltrated areas difficult to reach with a scalpel,

Aldara is a star. Applied directly to the tumor, the cream marshals the body's immune system to attack the cancer cells, which cannot then spread their evil tentacles any further. For patients with small, localized BCCs, Aldara provided a non-invasive and effective alternative to traditional surgery.

A patient applying the cream at home every couple of days for several weeks, with periodic checks from their dermatologist, may soon find that their skin, previously covered with lesions, returns to normal.

Beyond the Warts and Cancers – Treating Actinic Keratosis

There's another hidden treasure of Aldara: actinic keratosis. This is a condition where sun-damaged skin becomes precancerous. You might see scaly, rough patches that could, over time, turn into something more dangerous like skin cancer.

Aldara can't exactly reverse sun damage, but it helps in treating the precancerous cells, pushing the skin's immune system to take care of the abnormal growths.

Here, you get a case of an elderly man who loves his time in the sun but starts noticing these dry, irritating patches popping up on his skin. After a few treatments with Aldara, those patches begin to fade as his immune system does the heavy lifting.

CHAPTER TWO

Challenges and Side Effects – Not All Creams Are Created Equal

But of course, even something as powerful as Aldara has its challenges. Not everyone experiences the same results.

Some may experience intense irritation-redness, burning, swelling, and even flu-like symptoms during treatment. It's as if the immune system is overzealous in its work, sometimes overworking at the expense of the patient.

For example, say you have been treating a spot of actinic keratosis on your scalp. The skin underneath is sensitive, and suddenly you're experiencing a deep itch and inflammation. As your body starts to fight the abnormal cells, you may end up feeling a little like you overdid itworked out too hard, and your body aches. In just this way, the immune system can overreact to the added stimulation and cause temporary discomfort.

Fortunately, the irritation often subsides with continued use, and the effects taper down as the body continues its healing work.

The Fine Line – Compliance and Consistency

Aldara is not a "slap it on and forget about it" medication. It requires consistent application- usually, several weeks of regular use. Some patients don't take the treatment seriously, especially when the early signs of improvement show up. But stopping too soon can end the treatment prematurely, allowing the issue-be it warts or skin precancer-another chance to resurface.

Take, for example, a young man who's treating his genital warts. Weeks into the process, he sees improvement, and the warts shrink considerably. But then, unsure of whether the war is truly won, he decides to stop. A few weeks later, they returned. This cycle of starting and stopping can lead to greater frustration. The moral of the story? Consistent treatment is key, and doctors emphasize it to their patients at every opportunity.

Aldara and Its Companion Treatments

Oddly enough, Aldara often is used in combination with other treatments. In the case of genital warts, for example, Aldara is often prescribed in addition to other treatments such as cryotherapy or surgical removal for maximum effectiveness. By complementing Aldara's immune-boosting effects, doctors can ensure that warts don't just shrink but also don't come back post-treatment.

Similarly, in the management of basal cell carcinoma, surgeons may use Aldara after excision of a tumor in the hope of preventing its recurrence. There is power in combination when used sagaciously.

The Clinical Experience - Trials and Real-World Impact

Over the years, doctors across the globe have seen the effectiveness of Aldara in multiple clinical settings. For a dermatologist treating basal cell carcinoma, Aldara provides another tool in their arsenal to keep patients from having to undergo surgery. The process is simple: apply the cream on the designated area, wait, and monitor progress.

One oncologist related a story of a patient who had early-stage skin cancer and was apprehensive about surgery. They decided to try Aldara first. Several weeks into treatment, the affected area showed signs of improvement, and the patient avoided a big procedure—a win-win situation.

The Future of Aldara – Growing Beyond Expectations

The influence of Aldara doesn't stop with just one or two skin conditions. Researchers continue to find new ways that it could help in treating other skin cancers and immunologic conditions.

Some are even testing it on wound healing and scar tissue recovery, looking into exactly how Imiquimod may influence immune response in unique scenarios.

Furthermore, in a world continuing to fight the human

papilloma virus (HPV) and an impending basal cell carcinoma and actinic keratosis as a consequence of aging populations, the place of Aldara is secure, but there is still more to research.

Like all medical treatments, Aldara has its pros and cons, but its unique methodology for using the immune system to heal the body from within places it as one of the more interesting topical medications available today.

THE END